Advance Acclaim

"Hyaluronic acid is one of the most exciting anti-aging molecules today and now is available to everybody. *The Hyaluronic Acid Instant Face, Anti-Aging, Rejuvenation Miracle* brings this message of rejuvenation, based on real science, to millions of people worldwide who will benefit from this safe and effective anti-aging nutrient."

—*L. Stephen Coles, M.D., Ph.D., the world's leading researcher on super centenarians*

"I've personally used hyaluronic acid for my own joint health. And I recommend to my patients. HA is really quite a miracle compound for both your inner health and outer skin beauty and health. That's why all my patients definitely will benefit from this remarkable book."

—*Michael Loes, M.D., M.D.(H.), Sierra-Tucscon Hospital*

THE Hyaluronic Acid
INSTANT FACELIFT, ANTI-AGING, REJUVENATION
Miracle

*A COMPLETE GUIDE
to the World's Most Exciting
Anti-Aging Compound for
Flexible Joints, Vibrant Skin
and a Healthy Heart*

by
Dr. Chris Meletis
and
David Rousett

Disclaimer: This information is presented by an independent medical
expert whose sources of information include studies from the world's
medical and scientific literature, patient records, and other clinical and case
reports. The material in this book is for informational purposes only and is
not intended for the diagnosis, treatment, cure or prevention of disease.
Please visit a health professional for medical advice or to discuss
information contained in this book.

Book design by Bonnie Lambert.

ISBN 978-1-893910-69-0
Printed in the United States
Published by Freedom Press
120 North Topanga Canyon Boulevard
Topanga, CA 90290
Bulk Orders Available: (800) 959-9797
E-mail: info@freedompressonline.com

Table of Contents

1

Village of
Long Life

How would you like to live to one hundred years old without any of the aches and pains of aging, poor eyesight or dementia, without disease? Have you wanted to turn back on your aging skin? Do you want lines and wrinkles to disappear or an instant facelift? It sounds pretty good and there is a place where that might be possible.

Come visit Yuzuri Hara, the Village of Long Life, two hours outside of Tokyo, where people routinely live into their nineties without any of the usual signs of aging. In fact, more than ten percent of the villagers are 85 or older, ten times our national norm. The villagers enjoy excellent health, even though some of the villagers have unhealthy habits, such as smoking or unprotected sun exposure. Specifically, a 93-year-old farmer has worked in the fields in the sun for fifty years without once using the protection of sun block; yet, his skin is soft and smooth.

Cancer, diabetes, Alzheimer's—all are practically unheard of in this village.

The amazing anti-aging benefits of this miracle compound found in their diet were discovered only a few years ago.

The village is in a particularly hilly region, making rice cultivation difficult, so the people rely on raising a variety of starchy root vegetables. One of the major contributing factors to such circumstances is the high level of hyaluronic acid and its precursors available in these foods.

Like many of his peers who routinely live into their 90s and longer, Tadanao Takahashi was 93 at the time of the report and was in good health. Meanwhile, every morning, Hiroshi Sakamoto would wake up and farm his field, usually for about four or five hours a day. Sakamoto was 86 years old. But his age by no means made him the elder statesman of his village, nor is a daily routine like his uncommon among his peers.

These villagers have found the secret of long life in their traditional diet, which is unique. Unlike other regions of Japan that grow rice, Yuzuri Hara's hilly terrain is better suited to harvesting different carbohydrate-rich foods rich in sticky starches that may prove healthier: things like satsumaimo, a type of sweet potato; satoimo, a sticky white potato; konyaku, a gelatinous root vegetable concoction; and imoji, a potato root. These foods just happen to be rich in hyaluronic acid, and, as a result of their diet, the people of the village have higher levels of HA than most people have in their bodies.

This is a good thing. A very good thing. Many have even managed to keep their skin from showing signs of aging. The skin of people in their eighties and nineties feels like baby skin. Their eyesight is remarkable; most cannot remember a single day in which they were sick, even though many smoke. Doctors, farmers, innkeepers, all routinely practice their professions into their eighties.

The residents of Yuzuri Hara are not only living longer, but they are also quite healthy. Rarely do they have any reason to see a doctor. What makes the residents of Yuzuri Hara even more remarkable is that they are living long, healthy lives, even those who engage in unhealthy activities.

Sakamoto, for example, had smoked a pack and a half of cigarettes daily and was still in reasonably good health and physically fit. Takahashi had worked in the sun for 50 years, never once using sun block or skin cream, and yet his skin was soft and smooth. Japanese researchers think this phenomenon may be connected to the local diet.

The Secret Ingredient

Dr. Toyosuke Komori, the town doctor who has studied and written books on longevity in Yuzuri Hara, believes these locally grown starches help stimulate the body's natural creation of hyaluronic acid, which aging bodies typically lose. This may ward off the aging process by helping the cells of the body thrive and retain moisture, keeping joints lubricated, protecting the retina in eyes, and keeping skin smooth and elastic. "I have never seen anyone suffer from skin cancer here," he said. "I have seen a woman in her 90s with spotless skin." Komori, 80, who has adopted the local diet of very little meat and a lot of homegrown sticky starches, holds to his theory. "I feel very strongly that if I had not come here to Yuzuri Hara, I would not have lived this long and healthy of life," he said. "I probably would have died from some adult disease."

Komori also pointed to statistics showing that since Aging Western-style processed food infiltrated the village a few years ago, heart disease has doubled. With youngsters being seduced by these products, what the Japanese call an upside-down death pyramid has emerged, in which adults die before their elderly parents. "Although my children ate what I had been eating while they were young and lived here," says a 91-year-old woman who has outlived two of her six children, "when they moved away they chose to eat differently."

Fortunately, you don't have to visit Yuzuri Hara to take advantage of their longevity secret.

HA is available to consumers now that is virtually identical to the body's own HA and offers a perfect complement to HA injections given medical patients. Actually, both forms of HA are shown to be not only safe but to work in different but significant ways when it comes to anti-aging. In other words, all forms of HA—from injections to topical to oral even in shampoos, moisturizers and facial scrubs—are great! You want to give your body HA in all these forms.

So what is HA? That's a good question since it has only been in medical use here in the West since around 1997.

Hyaluronic acid is a carbohydrate, more specifically a mucopolysaccharide occurring naturally throughout the human body. HA loves to bind to water giving it a stiff viscous quality similar to "Jello." And it is the fact that this long-chained molecule loves water that appears to be why it is so good for our bodies.

This viscous gel is one of the most heavily researched substances in medicine today with thousands of clinical trials mostly in the fields of eye surgery and orthopedics where it used as a shock absorber to protect the retina or joints, respectively. Its function in the body is, among other duties, to bind water and to lubricate movable parts of the body, such as joints and muscles. HA's consistency and tissue-friendliness allows it to be used in skin-care products as an excellent moisturizer. It is one of the most hydrophilic (water-loving) molecules in nature and can be described as "nature's moisturizer."

The extracellular matrix (ECM) is a gel-like fluid that surrounds almost all living cells and is essential to life. It gives structure and support to the body and without it, we would just be a trillions cells without a shape or function. It is essentially the mortar between the bricks. The skin, bones, cartilage, tendons and ligaments are examples where the ECM is located in the body. The ECM is composed of material (fibrous elements) called elastin and collagen surrounded by gelatinous HA.

HA's roles in the ECM is to prevent the stretchy fibers in the body from overstretching and drying out by continually bathing them in this nutritious water-based gelatinous fluid. It also serves as a wonderful medium through which nutrients and waste are transported to and from the cells of these structures. This fluid would not exist if it was not for the ability of the HA molecule to bind up to 1000 times its weight in water.

But the most dramatic discoveries of HA's healing powers are just around the corner. After all, HA is integral to virtually all tissues and organs—and now medical science has proven that oral and topical HA is absorbable and beneficial—provided, of course, that you're using a high molecular weight non-animal source molecule with proven absorption and purity. (We'll give you some important shopping tips.)

Here are some of the most promising ways HA can benefit your quest to live as long and healthfully and as active, beautiful and handsome as possible.

Tendons and Ligaments/ Joints/Connective Tissue

HA is widely used now in joints since it supplies the synovial fluid that acts as a lubricant. You can ask your doctor about this alternative if you are experiencing such problems. But quite apart from injections, oral and topical HA also help a lot.

Eyes

Hyaluronic acid is a powerful eye tonic. No wonder, since HA is highly concentrated inside the eyeball. The fluid inside the eye called the vitreous humor is composed almost completely of hyaluronic acid. HA gives the fluid inside the eye a viscous gel like property. This gel acts as a shock absorber for the eye and also serves to transport nutrients into the eye.

Brain

Hyaluronic acid is a major part of the extracellular matrix of the brain, lending support to the vessels that supply the brain. It is thought that perhaps the deterioration of the brain seen in patients suffering from Alzheimer's disease, Parkinson's disease, senility, and stroke, could be, in part, due to the degradation of the vessels and the extracellular matrix. Likewise, perhaps this degradation could account for the shrinking of the brain seen in brain scans of people with advanced Alzheimer's disease.

Skin

Although HA can be found naturally in most every cell in the body, it is found in the greatest concentrations in the skin tissue. Almost fifty percent of the body's HA is found in skin tissue, both the deep underlying dermal areas as well as the visible epidermal top layers. As one of the skin's natural moisturizing elements, HA binds and holds water in the skin, enhancing the skin's elasticity. When this elasticity of the skin is lost, wrinkles form. The dermis of people over age sixty frequently contains no HA!

Gum Tissue

The gums (gingivoe) are composed of dense fibrous connective tissue (ligaments) which secure the teeth to the aveloar bone (jaw bone). Once again, connective tissue is composed of a fibrous tissue surrounded by hyaluronic acid (extra-cellular matrix). Without the hyaluronic acid, the gum tissue becomes unhealthy and may lead to swelling. If the HA is present it helps to provide the tensile strength of the ligaments that secure the tooth in place by providing hydration and nourishment. Regular use of HA helps to maintain a healthy set of gums.

Scalp Tissue and Hair Follicles

Actually the hair and the hair follicle are a derivative of skin tissue. There are two distinctive skin layers, one, the epidermis (outer layer), which gives rise to the protective shield of the body and the other, the dermal layer (deep layer), which makes up the bulk of the skin and is where the hair follicle is located. This dermal layer is composed of connective tissue and the connective tissue, with its gelatinous fluid like characteristics provides support, nourishes and hydrates the deep layers of the scalp. The result is healthy lustrous hair and a moisturized scalp. Again, all of this is made possible because of the presence of HA in the scalp tissue and its ability to form this fluid and hold water. No wonder consumers seek HA in shampoos and conditioners!

Lips

The lips are a core of skeletal muscle covered by skin tissue. The dermal layer of the lips is composed primarily of connective tissue and its components hyaluronic acid and collagen that give the structure (shape) and plumpness to the lips. The hyaluronic acid binds to water creating a gelatinous fluid that hydrates the surrounding tissue and keeps the collagen (responsible for keeping the skin tight) nourished and healthy. The result is healthy well hydrated and plump lips that are well protected from the environment.

EVER SINCE THE DISCOVERY of the miraculous benefits of HA in the village of Yuzuri Hara, this molecule has played a central role in many of the anti-aging strategies employed.

One approach is to make dietary changes, incorporating more magnesium, zinc, copper and silicon into our diet.

Another nutritional strategy is to favor foods and herbs that help the body prevent hyaluronidase, the enzyme that breaks down HA, from getting out of control and attacking our own valuable but scarce supplies.

We can visit a doctor for cosmetic HA treatments or to free ourselves from pain in an arthritic knee.

We can take oral high molecular weight (HMW) HA, use it in shampoos, conditioners, skin serums, scrubs, moisturizers, and other preparations.

These are powerful ways to battle the accumulative wear and tear that represents aging. You will learn about all of these approaches in the chapters that follow. We promise you that you will not only look but feel twenty years younger, thanks to HA. It really delivers.

It would make sense that the number-one water-binding molecule in nature, HA, would have to be linked with the process of anti-aging. It is, because it increases the "repair" part of the equation to offset and surpass the "wear and tear" portion. It's so easy to understand, anyone can apply it—and we do mean literally!

2

We all Need Lubricants and Shock Absorbers

How far would your car, truck, or lawnmower go without motor oil, transmission fluid, or steering fluid?

Machines need lubricants and shock absorbers—so do we!

These oils and fluids are essential for optimal performance. Their lubrication and shock-absorption abilities reduce friction and keep heat from building, which swells and destroys the engine parts. Just like machines, our bodies require lubrication and cushioning in order to move and do all we need to do each day.

The following is a brief overview of the many uses that hyaluronic acid has in the body:

1. If we deplete or break down the lubricating and shock-absorbing synovial fluid within our joints, we feel the heat of inflammation as the joints swell and grind against each other. Hyaluronic acid, or HA, is a crucial part of the synovial fluid that provides this lubrication.

2. The eye has a jellylike tissue within it known as the vitreous humor, which is the clear substrate that light shines through until hitting the back of the eye to form an image on the retina. The vitreous humor contains a large amount of hyaluronic acid that cushions the structures of the eye as we play contact sports, run, or just move about throughout the day. When this tissue breaks down due to a lack of HA, floaters occur as the degraded gel pulls free from the retina in a condition called posterior vitreous detachment, or PVD.

3. HA is critical to our arterial integrity and ability to transport nutrients in and out of organs; people with mitral valve prolapsed in their heart valves have had their body's HA destroyed by an enzyme called hyaluronidase produced by strep bacteria.

Going back to our machinery analogy, we see another similarity to the human body. Just as we use waxes and polymer treatments to keep a car's finish and upholstery in good condition, HA helps our skin remain in good condition. HA is a natural polymer, chemically made of many repeating units in a chain. By binding to 1,000 times its weight in water, HA and its attached water molecules plump the skin tissues to either fill in or prevent wrinkles, making skin look younger.

Beginning in 2003, the Food and Drug Adminsitration has approved hyaluronan injections for filling soft tissue defects such as facial wrinkles. These products are analogous to collagen injections but have the advantages of achieving longer lasting effects and decreasing the risk of allergic reactions. Hyaluronic acid is beneficial to the body for many reasons; as stated before, its decreased production can adversely affect bodily function. The Hyperhealth Database describes the correlation between HA production and aging: "The body's production of hyaluronic acid declines in tandem with the aging process and the body's excretion of hyaluronic acid increases in tandem with the aging process."

HA is used postoperatively to induce tissue healing, especially after cataract surgery. Large polymers of hyaluronic acid appear in the early stages of healing to physically make room for white blood cells involved in our immune response.

Methods to Ensure Optimal HA Levels in the Body

Fortunately, you can ensure optimal HA levels and activity in your body through a variety of strategies.

Below is a list of the various ways with a brief description of each.

Oral HA. Several varieties of oral HA supplements exist. There are low molecular weight HA supplements from animal sources and there are high molecular weight HA supplements with molecules that are 2–5 times longer than low molecular weight and there is bio-identical HMW HA which is about 5 times longer than high molecular weight. This bio-identical form exists in the same average length as the HA found within the body. Bio-identical HMW HA is vegan and is made through a process of natural fermentation. For our purposes, this is the preferred molecule that has been shown to be best absorbed and provide the desired benefits.

Topical Skin Care Ingredients. Citric acid and glycolic acid (both alpha hydroxyl acids), when applied topically, stimulate the development of HA in the skin, as does Retin-A. Coenzyme Q10 (CoQ10) applied topically increases the synthesis of HA within the skin in cells called fibroblasts. But your best source is pure bio-identical high molecular weight HA in combination with other key peptides, herbs and phytochemicals that will provide exactly the desired facial effect. That builds up the structure of your skin to provide your instant facelift. (See Chapter 6 for your instant facelift serum combinations.)

Injectable HA. Available from a medical doctor, HA injections can be performed on the skin, eye and joints. This type of pharmaceutical grade HA is usually of the high molecular weight variety.

HA Precursors. Some familiar compounds, such as glucosamine, chondroitin, N-acetyl glucosamine, shark cartilage and gelatin are involved in making HA while others aren't. These will be discussed later on in greater detail.

Hyaluronidase Inhibitors. Grape seed extract, green tea extract, quercetin, horse chestnut, and even some types of humectant, are examples of compounds that inhibit hyaluronidase, the enzyme that breaks down HA in the body. They are joined by various other bioflavonoids found within our diet and in capsules and tablets that will make your existing HA last longer.

Herbs. In addition to the plants mentioned above, gotu kola is legendary for its connective tissue building properties, aiding healing and enhancing brain function. It could be that gotu kola's effects on the body come from its ability to stimulate the production of endogenous (from within the body) HA levels.

Minerals. Zinc, magnesium, silicon, and copper contribute to building up HA levels.

Vitamins and Amino Acids. Vitamin C catalyzes the reaction that creates the connective tissue cousins of HA, collagen, and elastin. Vitamin C (ascorbic acid) is critical to HA production, so you want to be sure to consume citrus, peppers, and other rich in this nutrient. The amino acids converted into HA include proline and lysine.

3

Joint Health

To keep your automobile engine running smoothly you need to periodically replace the engine oil with new thick viscous oil, which certainly will keep it from breaking down for a very long time. Now the car has truly been fixed, not just treated. This is the same for using HA in one form or another). Whether people are using topical, oral or injectable HA, the results include the same great benefits that are just distributed in different ways. That's what makes HA so exciting. You don't need to go to the doctor for injections. Topical and oral HA are both great and deliver fantastic results.

A properly functioning joint allows for friction between cartilage using synovial fluid as a lubricant; this has been described as "ice on ice," a very slippery state, because it's similar to how an ice skater moves across the ice. The very thin metal blade of the ice skate creates so much force that a lubricating sheet of water forms directly beneath the skate. HA is a major portion of the synovial fluid that lubricates the joint capsule. Recent research has shown that the synovial fluid of patients with osteoarthritis has reduced levels of HA; logically, it seems that stimulating the production of more HA in these patients might be beneficial in the treatment of the disease.

Connective tissue is found everywhere in the body. It does much more than connect body parts; it has many forms and functions. Its major functions include binding, support, protection, and insulation. One such example of connective tissue is the cord-like structures that connect muscle to bone (tendons) and bone to bone (ligaments). In all connective tissue there are three structural elements. They are ground substance (hyaluronic acid), stretchy fibers (collagen and elastin) and a fundamental cell type. Whereas all other primary tissues in the body are composed mainly of living cells, connective tissues are composed largely of a nonliving ground substance (hyaluronic acid), which separates and cushions the living cells of the connective tissue. The separation and cushioning allow the tissue to bear weight, withstand great tension and endure abuses that no other body tissue could. All of this is made possible because of the presence of the HA and its ability to form the gelatinous ground substance fluid. No wonder studies with oral HA demonstrate excellent benefits for supporting joint health!

Hyaluronic acid is a special protein that is the normal lubricant in human joints. When present in a joint, even a joint with minimal or no cartilage, it can provide a cushion effect. Hyaluronic acid in our joints is a long complex molecule, and makes a ball shape which resists compression. However, with inflammation or other conditions the complex hyaluronic acid molecule breaks down to smaller pieces and is not effective in keeping a ball shape. Therefore it cannot provide a cushion of protection in the joint. Hyaluronic acid is also found in all connecting tissues of the body such as ligaments and tendons where it performs special functions of lubrication and helps orient ligament and tendon fibers.

Just as with osteoarthritis, sufferers of rheumatoid arthritis also have degraded HA in their synovial fluid. This is possibly due to the increased pressure within the joint capsule as tendons and ligaments strain against inflammation, causing increased friction that literally crushes the joint capsule.

Besides the high cost and inconvenience of injectable HA, the main difference between that and oral HA is that injectable HA is localized, while oral HA is delivered to the entire body. To expand on this topic, following are the results of studies performed on this comparison.

An April 2006 prospective study was conducted on 75 patients being treated for osteoarthritis of the ankle at the Department of Physical Medicine and Rehabilitation, Veterans General Hospital, Kaohsiung, Taiwan. After five weekly HA injections into the ankle joint, several objective measurements of joint health (assessed by orthopedic surgeons as well as by the patients' global satisfaction evaluation), including adverse events and consumption of rescue analgesics, were analyzed. Significant improvement in most of the objective measurements was noted at 1 week, 1 month, 3 months and 6 months past the fifth injection. Only range of motion of the joint didn't improve significantly. The patients reported 100% satisfaction at 1 week and 1 month, with 3-month scores of 90.7% and 6-month satisfaction scores rated at 86.7%. The clinical effect was rapid at 1 week and lasted for most patients for 6 months or more.

Similar results have been obtained with oral HA. In the six-month trial, called the "Oral Hyaluronic Acid Knee Arthritis Study" conducted by Dr. K.D. Reeves, a dosage level of two milligrams per day resulted in improvements in pain of 28 percent.

Dr. Reeves, a physician and medical researcher who holds a faculty appointment from the University of Kansas as Clinical Associate Professor in the Department of Physical Medicine and Rehabilitation, notes, "The literature continues to grow on the importance of hyaluronic acid in growth and repair.

"In summary, the two month data showed improvement in pain of 17% and 6 month data showed an improvement in pain of 28%," says Dr. Reeves. "The 6 month data is encouraging in that a placebo typically does not improve pain that much."

He says that the potential significance of oral hyaluronic acid is considerable and listed the following reasons:

It would represent a less invasive source of treatment.

It would potentially be less expensive than hyaluronic acid injections in the knee.

It would allow for avoidance of even the rare complication of joint infection or allergic reactions of delivery vehicles.

It is more convenient for the patient.

It may be advantageous by allowing for providing a convenient way whereby treatment can be delivered over a longer time frame than with inter-articular (directly into the knee) injections.

HA and Glucosamine

A lot of people already are using glucosamine sulfate or various other forms of glucosamine supplements. How do glucosamine and HA compare? Hyaluronic acid as an oral supplement has substantial differences from glucosamine sulfate. First, glucosamine is a modified simple sugar. Hyaluronic acid is a complex molecule with joint protective capability and a number of other properties that relate to its complexity. Although hyaluronic acid is complex, it is also 50% glucosamine, so that when it breaks down glucosamine is provided. That said, using both together is an excellent strategy.

Be sure when you use oral HA it is the bio-identical high molecular weight form. As we explain in our section on shopping for a great supplement, this is critical.

Also use topical HA, as found in moisturizing joint creams, which typically combine HA with cetyl myristoleate oil. Cetyl myristoleate (CM) was discovered back in 1964 by Harry W. Diehl, a chemist at the National Institutes of Health (NIH) in Bethesda, Maryland who was also instrumental in preparing a sugar for Dr. Jonas Salk's oral polio vaccination. Myristoleic acid occurs in minute quantities in all fats and oils and cetyl alcohol was originally obtained from the oil of sperm whales but now is derived from an environmentally friendly source, palmitic acid (a fatty acid in coconut and palm oils). As a result of his research, Diehl obtained two United States patents for demonstrating the potential of cetyl myristoleate in preventing and treating joint inflammation and pain. It seems to function in three ways: (1) It serves as a lubricant for the joints and muscles; (2) functions as an immune system modulator; and (3) acts as an anti-inflammatory agent by regulating prostaglandins, which are extremely potent mediators of inflammatory bodily processes.

Soaking in HA is also great for pain relieving and rejuvenating joints, ligaments, and tendons. Usually about 15 minutes is required for the HA to be taken up by your skin pores. Use a high quality soak without any toxic ingredients.

A moisturizinag joint soak with HA is a great choice. Its essential oils act as a carrier for the HA. There are many receptor sites for HA in the dermis so the HA is able to attach to these sites and be absorbed to provide soothing, moisturizing benefits.

HA and Athletes

HA can offer benefits to anyone who is subject to extended amounts of physical activity. In this case, HA should be combined with key nutrients to support muscle performance, power output, and normal recovery time after strenuous activity. L-carnosine is a dipeptide that binds to hydrogen ions as an intracellular buffer. Carnosine helps muscular pH by soaking up hydrogen ions (H+) that are released at an accelerated rate during exercise. The unique combination helps support the muscular and connective tissue systems as well as the joint and skeletal structures of the legs and joints. Due to the large amounts of stress on both of these systems when we are highly active, this is a smart way to build up your strength and resistance to injury, as well as work out harder and longer.

Connective Tissue Support

For anybody who is active or cares about their health, we get it that our tendons and ligaments also need to be strong. Powerful ingredients, such as hyaluronic acid, glutamine, n-acetyl glutamate, vitamin C, lysine and grape seed extract support healthy connective tissue and vessels. Glutamine is a major cellular energy source and the most abundant naturally occurring, non-essential amino acid in the human body. It can be found in the body's circulatory system and is stored in the skeletal muscles. N-Acetyl glucosamine, or NAG, is one of the eight main essential sugars the body needs for immune system health and overall body health. Several studies have shown that NAG aids in supporting healthy cartilage and ligament function, as well as digestive tract health. Vitamin C is an essential nutrient and antioxidant, responsible for manufacturing compounds necessary for healthy levels of HA in the body. L-lysine is an essential amino acid and protein builder and necessary for ligament health. Grape seed extract is a powerful antioxidant and inhibitor of hyaluronidase. The natural plant extract contains procyanidolic oligomers or more commonly known as PCO, known to maintain healthy bones and blood vessels as well as supports healthy blood circulation.

4

Heart and Circulatory Health

Do you think your arteries and blood vessels require adequate HA? You bet. Blood vessels, especially arteries and arterioles (small-sized branches of arteries), are unique in that they face the wear and tear from a pulsing pump (the heart) that beats over 100,000 beats per day on average. They expand and contract in response to the pulsing blood flow, and to control blood pressure.

One of the reasons that HA is so widespread in the body is that, in addition to its use in synovial fluid in the eyes and skin, it is one of the most important components of loose connective tissue that makes up the gel-like mortar between the cells that allows for the integrity of all our vessels—including our arteries and arterioles.

Water, salts, and other low-molecular-weight substances are contained within the extracellular matrix of the arteries but their main structural constituents are proteoglycans. The matrix is the connective tissue of the body (minus the collagen fibers, which are considered a separate entity).

Blood vessels are made up of HA-rich connective tissue. If the HA, collagen, and elastin in the blood vessels are weakened and compromised, arterial disease develops.

Dr. Mathias Rath, a leading researcher into the long-term health benefits of HA, notes, "Preserving and restoring the integrity and stability of the vascular wall is the most important therapeutic aim for prevention and treatment of human [coronary vascular disease]."

HA cushions the vessels with the water it attracts and drastically reduces the friction that would tear up your arteries within days. Is it any wonder that as we get older and lose HA, our skins grows more wrinkled, our joints get arthritis, and cardiovascular health can suffer heart attacks, peripheral artery disease, strokes and aneurysms?

Doctors can't inject your vessels with HA, but you can start a program to boost HA, collagen, and elastin levels, while slowing the detrimental effects of hyaluronidase, collagenase and elastase enzymes that break down and degrade HA and eventually contribute to the destruction of your pipes.

Remember having sufficient HA is critical for your body's 24-7 maintenance and repair program.

We recommend daily oral HA for supporting all of your connective tissues, including the arterial network. Be sure to increase your intake of ascorbic acid or vitamin C, which also stimulates the body's production, and to use inhibitors of hyaluronidase which breaks down the body's HA stores. Eat more citrus and peppers for your ascorbic acid, or take a quality supplement that provides all of the vitamin C synergists called flavonoids.

You should also consider combining HA with coenzymne Q10, one of the most intensively studied cardio nutrients. CoQ10 is a fat-soluble vitamin-like substance present in every cell of the body; it serves as a co-enzyme for several of the key enzymatic steps involved with cellular energy support and helps keep our heartbeat regular and strong. Resveratrol supports healthy blood flow and overall cardiovascular health and is a highly active polyphenol (a type of antioxidant) found in abundance in the skin of red grapes. Resveratrol helps our arteries to stay free from harmful plaque. Cranberry seed oil is rich in tocotrienols and tocopherols which are the two groups of molecules that make up vitamin E as well as other important antioxidants. The tocotrienols and tocopherols together are healthier than simply using alpha-tocopherol supplements. Studies have found that this oil contains the highest amount of tocotrienols than in any vegetable oil. Omega 3, 6, and 9 essential fatty acids, not found in any other oil, are also unique to cranberry seed oil. It is rich in vitamin A, is a great alternative to fish oil and has a very stable shelf life. Choosing a comprehensive supplement, including some of the key ingredients above,will provide you with antioxidant protection, support healthy cholesterol levels, and help you maintain already healthy blood pressure levels, besides helping to maintain the structural integrity of your arterial's tissues.

In addition to your core HA heart health supplement which you will want to take every day you should combine your supplement with grape seed and green tea together with quercetin, and horse chestnut, compounds that inhibit hyaluronidase, the enzyme that breaks down HA in the body. These are some of the most powerful flavonoid-rich compounds to use for maintaining healthy HA levels in your body. Again, seek quality supplements.

Be sure to include gotu kola with your HA program. Gotu kola is legendary for its connective tissue building properties, aiding healing and enhancing brain function. How does gotu kola exert its remarkable wound healing effects? Studies show it helps the body to maintain healthy connective tissues by maintaining the vessels that enable the blood to reach them. Gotu kola also helps the body manufacture structural substances such as hyaluronic acid, a viscous medium in the body, and chondroitin sulfates which also help to impart shape to the body's structural tissues. At the same time, gotu kola's effects on fibroblasts which contribute to the formation of connective tissues help to reduce sclerosis or hardening of the tissues.

Be sure you have adequate trace minerals via coral minerals, algae-based calcium or other complete sources. The minerals zinc, magnesium, silicon, and copper contribute in building up HA levels.

Vitamin C catalyzes the reaction that creates the connective tissue cousins of HA, collagen, and elastin. The compounds that are converted are the amino acids proline and lysine.

Helps Varicose and Spider Veins

A look at the cause of varicose veins, spider veins, and hemorrhoids shows a very close similarity to the underlying need for healthy arterial tissues. The squeezing of leg muscles pumps blood back to the heart from the lower body. When we sit for extended periods, especially on hard surfaces, we take these leg pumps "out of the game." Veins have valves that act as one-way flaps. These valves prevent the blood from flowing backwards as it moves up the legs. If the one-way valves become weak, blood can leak back into the vein and collect there. This problem is called venous insufficiency. Pooled blood enlarges the vein and it becomes varicose. Spider veins can also be caused by the backup of blood. These valves fail because excess pressure meets valves containing degraded HA and collagen.

Once again, deal with your connective tissue problems with a diet that enhances connective tissue issues as you will now for overall health and take bio-identical high molecular weight HA orally, and additionally apply bio-identical HA with horse chestnut to the skin from a HMW serum or lotion. Also, take varicose vein formulas that include horse chestnut to support vein health and grape seed extract to help control the effects of hyaluronidase.

Varicose veins are the most common of venous system diseases. The condition appears to increase with age and shows little gender bias. If left untreated, varicose veins can lead to leg eczema and ulcers. Occasionally, symptoms of this disease can lead to hospitalization and/or early retirement.

The enzyme hyaluronidase increases permeability of the veins, which promotes further venous insufficiency. Hyaluronidase also facilitates growth of the smooth muscle cells, which contribute to varicose veins. Horse chestnut's escin inhibits hyaluronidase. This allows cells lining the veins to better tolerate a lack of oxygen. This breaks the vicious circle of venous insufficiency, leading to less inflammation, less swelling, and fewer white blood cells accumulating. In theory, use of horse chestnut seed should also lead to less vein growth and less varicose veins, though this has not been tested directly.

The addition of curcumin-rich turmeric should also help to inhibit growth factors that enable the cells of the veins to continue to grow and lose more integrity. Grape seed extract helps to restore the integrity of the veins too. So do look for these ingredients in topical formulas.

From grape seed to horse chestnut, curcumin and vitamin C, these are all good supplements to take, especially when combined with bio-identical HMW HA.

5

Eyes and
Nervous System

C*an hyaluronic acid affect your eyesight? With the right sup-*
plement, the answer is yes.

The saying "the eyes are the windows to the soul" has been
around nearly since the beginning of recorded time. Variously at-
tributed to the bible (Matthew 6:22-23) and to the Roman statesman Cicero (106-43 B.C.), it has come to symbolize clarity.
Imagine, then, if the windows were cloudy. The ability to see the
world clearly would be greatly diminished. Luckily, the eyes of the
world have a great window washer in hyaluronic acid.

Hyaluronic acid makes up 95 percent of the fluid inside the
eye. It acts as a shock absorber as well as a nutrient transportation
device, and it helps play a major role in maintaining the health of
ocular tissues like the cornea, retina and the vitreous fluid that
fills the inside of the eye. Poor vision, linked to aging and increased exposure to harmful environmental factors, has also been
linked to a lack of nutrients that support healthy, clear and bright

eyes. A six-year clinical evaluation on hyaluronic acid, published in the *Archives of Ophthalmology* (1979;97;12:2325-30), showed that it was well-tolerated by human eyes. In fact, in eyes that had been given a poor prognosis, hyaluronic acid was helpful in preserving corneal integrity and clarity. In addition, in Japan, where hyaluronic acid-rich starches are consumed, people enjoy unusually healthy eyesight into their eighties and nineties.

According to a national public health strategy report on vision problems, prepared by Prevent Blindness America (in collaboration with the American Academy of Ophthalmology, American Optometric Association, Lighthouse International and National Alliance for Eye and Vision Research) an estimated 80 million people have a potentially blinding eye disease, three million have low vision, 1.1 million are legally blind and some 200,000 are severely visually impaired. One of their goals is to educate the general public on maintaining vision health, something greatly needed.

Supplements for Eye Health

The human eye is the only place in the body where both the nerves and blood vessels of the body can be fully visualized without cutting into the body. The eyes literally act as a window to the status of your health. With macular degeneration, diabetes, and high blood pressure leading to an ever-increasing number of people to lose some or all of their vision, now is the time to take charge.

It is imperative to be proactive when it comes to your health, especially your eyes. After all, when you become forced to be reactive in the arena of health, you are already behind and are trying to play catch up to regain your health, rather than more simply maintaining it.

Along with hyaluronic acid, some of the most important elements for eye health are lutein and zeaxanthin. These antioxidants are compounds called xanthophylls. They're found in large amounts in the lens and retina of our eyes, helping provide protection from damage caused by unstable free radicals. Lutein and zeaxanthin may also help protect eyes by filtering high-energy blue light. A February 2001 study between Johns Hopkins University and the Chinese University of Hong Kong indicated that these two ingredients act almost like sunglasses, protecting the retina and the macula.

Other nutrients vital to healthy eyesight include bilberry, to promote healthy eye circulation, improve night vision and prevent eyestrain.

In one study, bilberry extract together with vitamin E halted cataract progression in 97 percent of 50 patients with cataracts.[i] Grape seed extract is very protective against some forms of ultraviolet radiation.[ii]

Vitamins A, C and E are also positive influences on eye health, as is zinc which helps your body absorb these powerful antioxidants. The National Eye Institute's Age-Related Eye Disease Study (AREDS) recently stated that the "high doses achieved with supplementation appear to provide protective effects against the progression of macular degeneration."

Some of the most exciting and well-proven nutrients for cataract prevention are vitamins C and E, beta-carotene and other members of the carotene family, and the mineral selenium. These nutrients appear to protect the tissues of the eye from damage caused by the ultraviolet rays of the sun. In fact, there is some evidence that carotenes, such as beta-carotene, work like filters to protect the lens.[iii]

Based on many epidemiological and case-control studies, we know that persons who have the highest dietary intakes or circulating blood levels of these nutrients tend to have much lower risks for developing cataracts.[iv, v]

Certainly, it is important to eat foods rich in these nutrients: citrus, peppers, carrots, leafy green vegetables (e.g., spinach), and whole grains.

And, of course, no eye care program would be complete without HA. In fact, one of the best sources of eye health is high molecular weight hyaluronic acid, or HA, a major component of the eye and thus its visionary health. It's HA that gives the fluid inside the eyes its viscous gel-like property. Once we enter into our 50s, and sometimes before, our eyes stop producing hyaluronic acid, a condition that leads to poor vision, dry eyes and other potential problems.

Eye surgeons inject HA directly into the eye to help maintain the shape of the eye during surgery. It has been said that after the fifth decade of life, our eyes stop producing the much needed hyaluronic acid resulting in various eye problems such as poor vision, dry eyes, and floaters. Today, oral and topical HA are also thought to help support ocular health, particularly based on proprietary research in Japan on HA pills in which users reported improved vision.

What Does HA Do for the Eyes?

In the eye, HA acts as a shock absorber and lubricant and keeps the structures of the eye snug so that they work optimally. Think of how different it feels to walk barefoot on a hard surface—you can feel the shock in your legs and hips—versus walking with soft shoes or cushioned insoles. Most of this skeletal shock is transferred up the vertebral column to the skull and the eyes and brain. It only makes sense to have a shock absorber within the eyes to stabilize vision and protect delicate eye tissues. As in the joints, HA also helps aid transport of nutrients. Hyaluronic acid in the eye is found in a structure called the vitreous humor, which is a clear gel that fills the central part of the eye.

It's formed by a network of collagen and HA and occupies about 80 percent of the eyeball's volume. The hyaluronic acid molecules are large coils that hold water; in the vitreous they are entrapped in a matrix of collagen fibers. Most of the collagen is at the surface region of the vitreous, where it comes in contact with the rest of the eye, giving it a somewhat more solid surface. There is less collagen in the central region, which is a more liquid portion, comprised of about 99 percent water. Collagen fibrils attach the vitreous gel to points around its margin, particularly to the retinal and lens structures.

Floaters

The original three-dimensional net-like structure of collagen fibers begins to deteriorate once body growth has halted at adolescence. This deterioration is slow and involves having some strands of collagen clump up, and some of the original compartments of gel merge into larger compartments. At this point, "floaters" may begin to appear, usually in people between 40 and 70 years of age, but can occur earlier in the nearsighted or those that have undergone cataract surgery. Many people believe that these floaters are materials released into the eye, when, in fact, they are shadows on the retina from light encountering the irregularities in the gel matrix. Such irregularities are mainly caused by coalesced collagen filaments, which form fibrils. The floaters are especially visible while looking at a plain, well-lit background. Floaters look like spots, dots, or curly lines that move with your eye and appear suspended in front of you. Flashes of light are also a common eye complaint, a symptom of posterior vitreal detachment (PVD), and are produced from the pulling on the retinal tissue as the gel separates. The pulling fires the nerves on the retina, producing a flashing image. In serious PVD where a retinal hemorrhage occurs, people see a shower of sparks. Large hemorrhages can produce large blobs in the field of vision and you could even suffer a retinal tear which can be much more serious since the vitreous can get behind the tear, pushing even more retinal tissue loose. Most PVDs aren't associated with retinal tears, but one thing's for sure, there's a correlation between the breakdown of HA within the vitreous and the breakdown of intercellular HA in the dermis, the vessels, and the synovial fluid. An HA protocol should be started to produce more new HA within the vitreous and throughout the body.

HA and the Nervous System

The human brain is dynamic and is without question the most amazing suspended mass of cells ever created. The 100 billion neurons (cells) that comprise the human brain are the composite of tissue types, including solid matrix, and water, and weighs a total of about 3 pounds (approximately 2 percent of a 150-pound person).Yet the maintenance of the adult human brain demands 20 percent of oxygen delivery from each heartbeat. It is maintaining that high energy that requires the proper structural integrity be sustained. There is a saying that structure begets function and function begets structure. Well, without sufficient structural integrity, the brain won't work (just as an egg beater that doesn't have all its parts solidly in place would not function up to expectations).

The brain is supported structurally to a great extent by HA; this is important since HA is responsible for maintaining the massive 77 percent water content. Now that is what you can call structured water! There is very little collagen within the brain, but HA is there in quantity, as is chondroitin sulfate. Hyaluronic acid plays the main structural role in the formation of the brain's extracellular matrix (ECM). The extracellular space appears empty by elec-

tron microscopy because HA is readily soluble during the prepa-
ration of tissues for ultra structural studies. Cells containing HA
are found in many areas of the brain. It is noteworthy to point out
that HA-containing neurons were not significantly altered in
Alzheimer's disease (AD) patient's brain, suggesting that these
neurons are resistant to the pathological process of AD. When a
stroke occurs as a result of a clot, causing ischemia (lack of sufficient blood flow) or infarction (stoppage of blood flow), much of
the damage is to the structural integrity of the brain and to its
blood vessels, partly through the release of matrix metallopro-
teases, enzymes that break down hyaluronic acid and other elements of connective tissue. Other proteases also contribute to this
process. The loss of vascular structural integrity results in a breakdown of the protective blood brain barrier that contributes to
cerebral edema, which can cause secondary progression of the
brain injury. The reality is that each moment, we are losing one
brain cell per second under the best circumstances. In order to
protect against accelerated brain damage and loss of brain integrity, it is important to remember that we are all experiencing,
through the aging process, the proverbial plum-to-prune, grape-
to-raisin transformation. After all what do we associate with
aging? That's right—wrinkling. Just like skin, the human brain is
also prone to shrinkage as it ages, and there is no question that
dehydration leads to cognitive decline. Who knew HA might be
good for cognitive health?

6

The HA
Instant Facelift
Miracle

Americans spent just under $12.5 billion on cosmetic procedures in 2004. There were nearly 11.9 million surgical and nonsurgical cosmetic procedures performed in 2004, according to the most comprehensive survey to date of U.S. physicians and surgeons by the American Society for Aesthetic Plastic Surgery (ASAPS). Surgical procedures represented 18 percent of the total, and nonsurgical procedures were 82 percent of the total. From 2003-2004, there was a 44 percent increase in the total number of cosmetic procedures. Since 1997, there has been a 465 percent increase in the total number of cosmetic procedures. Over 882,000 HMW HA (bio-identical) procedures were performed in 2004 alone! And studies show that the women and some men who received them loved them! When it comes to your skin, HA is your absolute best friend. Women rave that HA serums actually save them money by replacing the need for Botox sessions. Other women say that with HA serum they no longer feel the need for a surgical approach. Well, before you go to the surgeon, HA will give you an instant facelift.

It is known that aging causes increased dryness of skin, so it's no surprise that HA content of the body goes down as we age, resulting in drier skin, drier joints, shrunken organs (including the brain), and drier eyes. Its humectants feature is truly one of the reasons why HA is such a workhorse in the body.

Young skin is smooth and elastic and contains large amounts of HA that helps keep the skin stay young and healthy. The HA provides continuous moisture to the skin by binding up to 1000 times its weight in water. With age, the ability of the skin to produce HA decreases leaving the skin unhealthy and wrinkled. That's why topically applied HA is such a powerful anti-aging cosmeceutical.

The skin is the largest organ in the body, comprising about 15 percent of the body weight. The total skin surface of an adult ranges from one and a half to two square meters. Half of the body's HA is found in the skin in the dermis and epidermis layers. The skin is a mirror of an individual's state of health. A skin condition often reflects a deeper state of imbalance.

What Happens to Our Skin as We Age?

Young skin is smooth and elastic and contains a large amount of hyaluronic acid that helps the skin look healthy. As we grow older, the ability of the skin to produce hyaluronic acid decreases and the amount of hyaluronic acid begins to fall. Since hyaluronic acid helps to bind water, the ability of the skin to retain water also declines with age. As a result, the skin becomes drier, thinner, and less able to restore itself. The loss of skin fullness also means that the skin becomes looser. This leads to wrinkling and the older appearance of the skin.

The skin consists of three main layers: the epidermis, dermis and subcutaneous tissue. The epidermis is the outer layer that protects our bodies from heat and cold. The condition of the epidermis determines how the skin looks and also how well the skin absorbs and holds moisture. Wrinkles, however, are formed in lower layers. The dermis is the middle layer of the skin and the skin's support structure. It is the thickest layer and comprises a network of collagen and elastin fibers. The subcutaneous tissue consists mainly of fat that keeps the body warm, stores energy, and protects inner organs. The dermis represents 90 percent of the thickness of the skin (the epidermis above it makes up the other 10 percent). Collagen makes up 70 percent of the dry weight of the dermis. The dry part is the key, since HA hydrates the dermis so effectively that it is about 70 percent water, representing 15-18 percent of the total body water. Hyaluronic acid within the dermis normally hydrates it, providing elasticity to prevent wrinkles. Since HA chemically attracts water, topical HA (as well as oral) can help by increasing endogenous HA in the dermis or by attracting a water layer on top of the skin surface to protect against water loss.

In the May 2008 issue of the *Dermatologic Surgery* journal, researchers commented on HA's ability to rejuvenate facial skin. They observed that skin changes associated with aging, such as loss of elasticity and roughening, have a negative psychosocial impact. In other words, we are all fighting the battle of aging! Elasticity, skin surface roughness, dermal thickness and density were evaluated at each treatment session and at 4 and 12 weeks after the last treatment session. "During the course of the study, skin elasticity and surface roughness improved significantly. Patient feedback was extremely positive." Conclusion? HA "can exert a rejuvenating effect on facial skin."

Significant Results in Favor of Vegan HMW Hyaluronic Acid

In a clinical study that compared HMW HA with a collagen-based product in 138 patients, six times as many patients found better effects with HMW HA than those that received collagen.

Before (top) and after (bottom) effects of patients having received injections of HMW HA.

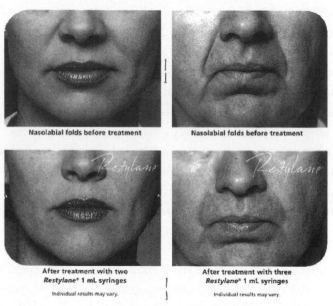

Courtesy Medicis/Restylane

Bio-identical HA Promising in Facial Soft-Tissue Augmentation

In a randomized, patient- and evaluator-blinded study, 150 patients seeking treatment for the correction of nasolabial folds were given HMW HA and a competing product (with low molecular weight hyaluronic acid derived from rooster combs) on opposite sides of the face. The study revealed that HMW HA produced a more durable aesthetic improvement than the competing product in 57 percent of the patients after six months and that fewer treatment sessions were needed to obtain an optimal result with HMW HA than the other LMW HA product.

However, quite apart from injections, topical HA offers truly amazing benefits. A former model says that she would not go a day without HA because it provides an instant facelift and removes the lines that so many celebrities are visiting their doctors for to have Botox treatment. Because they work so well and are formulated with purity and potency for your instant facelift, there is a particular brand available at health food stores, natural pharmacies, and spas that we strongly recommend you use for topical HA (see Resources). Each of these formulas complements bio-identical HMW HA with clinically studied phytochemicals and peptides—and they work extremely well. Here's what we recommend when it comes to combinations to address specific beauty issues.

Instant Facelift Serum with Peptides

Use Instant Facelift Serum for your instant facelift. Instant Facelift Serum is an effective combination of HA and proprietary peptides designed to hydrate and support the natural firmness and elasticity of the skin. The tightening peptide complex in the formula is a unique ingredient with the ability to support the skin's natural firmness and vitality. It is derived from a microalgae and designed to firm and tighten skin while at the same time promoting a healthy collagen network.

This algae/polysaccharide blend tightens the skin while protecting sensitive tissues against oxidative stress, a major contributor to skin aging. This peptide complex significantly reduces oxidative stress in skin cell cultures. With this formula you will lift and and tighten loose skin. The efficacy of the peptide complex in this formula was performed in a study with 30 volunteers during 2 weeks that demonstrated a very good and tightening effect, as you can see from the chart below in figure one.

Figure One:
Clinical Trial Results

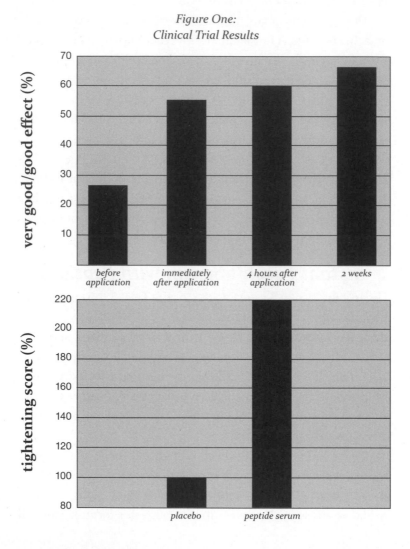

Facial Relaxation Serum

Want to avoid Botox treatments? Try Facial Relaxation (also known as FRS) Serum, a powerful combination of HA and Argireline® designed to hydrate, nourish and relax expression lines to lessen the appearance of wrinkles. Argireline® is a unique hexapeptide that has been shown to relax and smooth expression lines around the eyes, forehead and mouth to lessen the appearance of wrinkles.

If you have "worry" lines marring your skin, see for yourself what this miracle combination can do for you! Argireline (acetyl-hexapeptide-3) relaxes the facial muscles that are responsible for expression lines and wrinkles. Researchers think Argireline works by inhibiting the release of neurotransmitters released by the brain that tell these facial muscles to tense. The result is relaxed musculature and reduced wrinkles and lines. Note that Argireline's effects are very similar to those of Botox injections; however, where the FDA allows Botox serum to be injected in limited areas of the face, Argireline may be applied wherever lines and wrinkles appear. One published study showed a nearly 30 percent reduction in wrinkle size after only 30 days of using Argireline. Skin topography analyses were performed by obtaining silicon imprints

Figure Two:
Argireline Facial Relaxation Study Results

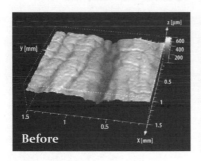 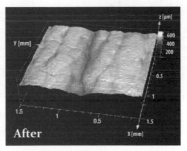

from around the eyes of 10 healthy women volunteers. Skin topography images from the three dimensional reconstruction of optical sections are shown in figure two. The depth of the wrinkle decreased an average of 27%, with maximum values between 50 and 60%.

Age Defense

An effective combination of HA and coenzyme Q10 (CoQ10) designed to hydrate, nourish and rejuvenate your skin, CoQ10 is found in every cell of the body and helps maintain healthy skin re-

Figure Three:
CoQ10 Wrinkle Reduction Study Results

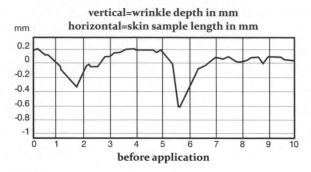

before application

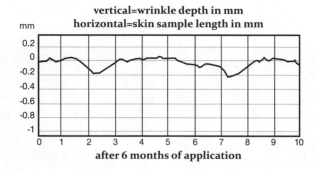

after 6 months of application

From BioFactors 9 (1999) 371-378, IOS

newal. It nourishes and protects the skin. In a 1999 study published in *Biofactors* done over a six-month period that examined the effects of CoQ10 on 20 elderly volunteers once daily around the eyes for six months, researchers observed a 27% reduction in wrinkles, as shown in figure three below.

Dark Circle Lightener Serum

Dark Circle Lightener (DCL) serum combines HA with two new plant-based peptide ingredients (Eyeseryl® and Regu®Age) designed to hydrate your skin and lighten the appearance of dark eye circles. Together these peptides dramatically reduce dark circles and unsightly puffiness around the eyes. They also reduce the microcirculation and the proteolytic breakdown of the collagen and elastin matrix. Dark circles and puffiness may be caused by the pooling of blood and a decrease in the strength of the skin's collagen network. These ingredients help to nourish and revive the skin, which can help you look your very best.

Figure Four:
CLINICAL RESEARCH

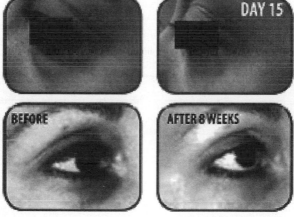

The exciting new ingredients in this serum can help to lessen the appearance of dark circles while restoring a healthy skin tone and color under the eyes.

In the top results, testing was done on 20 volunteers and the serum was applied twice a day for 60 days. Seventy percent of the volunteers had improved in only 15 days with 95% reporting improvement by the end of 60 days .

In the bottom before and after picture, testing was done on 20 volunteers and the serum was applied twice a day for 8 weeks. The study was performed on a double blind randomized basis.

Age Spot Lightener

Age Spot Lightener (ASL) Serum is an effective combination designed to hydrate your skin while lightening and toning age spots. HA, combined with a blend of seven alpine plants, is shown to reduce the color and intensity of age spots while regulating skin tone, as shown in figure five.

In a clinical study, the herbal complex showed significant lightening activity after 12 weeks of treatment without observing any particular irritation. It also "shows significant reduction of age-spots color intensity."

Figure Five:
GIGAWHITE™ SKIN LIGHTENING STUDIES

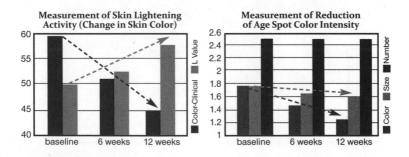

Pore Minimizer

Finally, there is a new skin care formula that we see on the market for teens and adults, who are looking for an all-natural product to control shine and oiliness, as well as improve the look, feel and texture of their skin, using the patented cleansing properties of Regu®-Seb, while providing rejuvenating antioxidants. Hyaluronic acid and green tea extract have been added to soothe and moisturize, leaving skin smooth and fresh all day.

A key ingredient is Regu®-Seb, an ivory, slightly viscous solution made of several fruit extracts that contain high levels of natural lignans and phytosterols. It contains polyphenol-rich fractions from the fruits of the North American saw palmetto and South American sesame seeds in a Moroccan argan oil base. With a perfectly balanced polyphenol formula, it helps to control and reduce sebum production, especially in the T-zone area of the face.

In one study, a significant decrease of 46% in sebum skin production was shown. Skin appearance was improved.

Benefits for most HA formulas typically occur in as little as two weeks, although some will notice benefits within one week. The most dramatic performance benefits are generally experienced within the 3-4 week range but they don't stop there. (Of course, this presumes one is using high molecular weight bio-identical HA. Other lower molecular weight HA products have other benefits but not those associated with anti-aging and a healthy inflammation and pain response).

No doubt, HA will be seen in many more formulas as the scientific evidence for its health benefits mounts and its popularity increases. It truly is a miracle for staying active and maintaining beautiful ageless skin.

How to Use HA Serum

Please keep in mind most of the studies here are showing great results with simply topical applications. You can safely use HA injections under a qualified doctor's supervision but you can get all the benefits of HA and other key peptides with topicals, too. Apply twice a day to wet skin or put a small amount on the back or side of your hand, and mix with an equal amount of water. These serums are very concentrated and adding a very small amount of water will help activate them for best results. Apply to the areas you desire to see results according to the serum you choose!

But one thing we do know: use these before you contemplate surgery or Botox treatment. You will be amazed at the fact that you probably won't need either!

7

HA in Medicine and Nutrition

As of 2006, the most widely used type of injectable, HA-based fillers is non-animal stabilized hyaluronic acid (NASHA).

Two of the best-known injectable brands are Restylane® and Captique®.

NASHA is made in a rather sophisticated way. Bioengineered bacteria produce HA that is nearly identical to that found in human skin. NASHA is then purified and treated with a cross-linking agent, which converts it into a stable, firm gel. Finally, the HA gel is dispersed in microspheres to make it easily injectable. Depending on the degree of cross-linking and the size of the microspheres, the products are used for different cosmetic purposes. One type is for moderate wrinkles and lip enhancement. Another is for deep lines, facial contouring, and lip enhancement. Yet a third type is for very thin superficial lines. A SubQ type is designed to replace fat loss in the face and create or restore a more defined facial contour.

NASHA costs around $500-$600 per cc (cubic centimeter). A typical amount per treatment is from 3/4 to 2 cc ($375-$1,200). To maintain results, the treatment has to be repeated every 6-12 months. The HA-based fillers of animal origin tend to be about 20-30 percent less expensive than NASHA. Some experts maintain that they are less durable than NASHA. Really, there isn't enough published data for a good durability comparison.

If you have osteoarthritis, the level of HA in your joint fluid is lower. So the joint fluid is less protective because it's thinner and less sticky. Three slightly different types of manufactured HA are available for the knee and osteoarthritis: Check with your doctor to find out which is right for you.

Oral and Topical Supplements

Because of the high cost of injections, many consumers are opting to use oral and topical HA formulas. We think this is great. As we say HA in any form is beneficial.

But you must be sure to purchase bio-identical high molecular weight HA like the kind used in the medical applications. This is by far the superior form of HA.

You will see cheaper products, but do not be fooled. Much has been made of new low molecular weight (LMW) HA from collagen type II. We've seen this type of HA in many different preparations, but we think your money would be better invested in bio-identical HA that is prepared in a similar manner to the HA that doctors use in injections. We're sure there are some benefits to low molecular weight preparations and they may even be absorbed better. The problem is, however, that they aren't as viscous (thick), so they don't hold water as well—remember, bio-identical HA holds over one thousand times its weight in water— to hydrate your skin, cushion your joints and eyes, and facilitate the transport of nutrients, toxins, and gases through the loose connective tissues of your body. The high molecular weight has all the "reeds" necessary to hold in water.

Also, low molecular weight HA looks less expensive, is only about 9-12 percent pure HA, so you get less HA per ounce. Bio-identical HA has over 90 percent HA in each dose. A lower dose of bio-identical HA delivers more of the fully functional form like that used in the body.

Buying LMW HA is like buying motor oil with the consistency of water just because it pours into the oil filler cap easier. Don't do this to your own body. Stay with the quality and proven form of HA and you will receive the amazing benefits we have told you about.

8

The HA Diet and Supplement Program

As we age, the enzymes that breakdown connective tissues (hyaluronidase, collagenase and elastase) are overexpressed, while our ability to make more HA decreases.

Grape seed extract's oligopolymers, green tea's catechins, and sulfur inhibit these enzymes enough for the body to reach equilibrium. That is why we highly recommend that people enjoy green tea and consider taking supplements such as grape seed and methylsulfonylmethane or MSM, a rich sulfur source.

Grape seed inhibits the activity of hyaluronidase. Grape seed can help combat atherosclerosis, ischemic heart disease, heart attacks, varicose veins, hemorrhoids, venous insufficiency, stroke, various types of cancer, diabetic retinopathy, and bloodshot eyes; this is thought to be due to powerful antioxidant effects.

However, in our opinion, it's more closely related to the fact that the phytochemicals from grape seed are the enemy of excess hyaluronidase, collagenase and elastase.

Green tea catechins are the polyphenol compounds responsible for most of green tea's beneficial actions. Sometimes they are referred to by their isomer variations, epicatechin, epicatechin gallate, epigallocatechin, epigallo- catechin gallate, or ECGC. They inhibit the destructive enzymes, too.

MSM, of course, is well known for helping people who have to deal with joint pain. This is thought to be due to its release of elemental sulfur, which also inhibits destructive enzyme activity.

Glucosamine is a constituent of HA (in the N-acetyl glucosamine form), and studies have shown that it is superior to ibuprofen as a painkiller after about 6 weeks of use. Why? Basically, ibuprofen and other NSAIDs (non-steroidal anti-inflammatory drugs) cut the wires (nerves) that deliver pain signals. Only the symptom (pain) is being treated; the joints are still breaking down, only you no longer feel it. Recent data also point to the fact that these NSAIDs, like ibuprofen and aspirin, actually damage joint tissues. Glucosamine (especially glucosamine sulfate) helps rebuild the joint tissues, restoring the cushion and, over time, lessening the pain as the joint is rebuilt. Together with HA's ability to reduce friction by building the synovial fluid that lubricates the joint, the joint can be restored.

Magnesium is a key mineral used by the body to build and maintain HA levels. "There's no question that magnesium is the most looked-at mineral in nutrition today," says Herbert C. Mansmann Jr., M.D., professor of pediatrics and associate professor of medicine at Jefferson Medical College of Thomas Jefferson University in Philadelphia. And the more research that's done, the better magnesium looks. Inside your body, magnesium serves several crucial roles, including helping to turn food into energy and assisting in the transmission of electrical impulses across nerves and muscles. These impulses generate what's called neuromuscular contraction—literally, causing your muscles to flex. Take magnesium away, and muscles, even the smooth muscles that routinely squeeze blood vessels, will cramp. That's one reason why an Epsom salt bath (originally from Epsom, England) relaxes you and takes away muscle tension. Epsom salt is made up of magnesium sulfate, providing both sulfur and magnesium to the body through the skin. Good food sources of magnesium are: avocados, bananas, broccoli, brown rice, haddock, navy beans, oatmeal, pinto beans, spinach, sweet potatoes, and yogurt.

Incorporating these foods into our diet is important since over 80% of us are low in magnesium.

Do you notice we listed sweet potatoes? This is a North American version of one of the root vegetables eaten by the Yuzuri- Harans, the long-lived people in mountainous Japan. Yuzuri Hara's hilly terrain is better suited to harvesting different carbohydrates that may prove healthier. Dr. Toyosuke Komori, the town doctor who has studied and written books on longevity in Yuzuri Hara, believes these locally grown starches help stimulate the body's natural creation of HA, which aging bodies typically lose.

Stocks and Broths Are Good for Your HA Levels

A sad outcome of our modern meat-processing techniques and hurry-up, throw-away lifestyle has been a decline in the use of meat, poultry, and fish stocks. Thirty or more years ago, when the butcher sold meat on the bone rather than as individual fillets, and whole chickens rather than boneless breasts, our thrifty ancestors made use of every part of the animal by preparing stock, broth, or bouillon from the bony portions. Meat and fish stocks are used almost universally in traditional cuisines: French, Italian, Chinese, Japanese, African, South American, Middle Eastern, and Russian. However, the use of homemade meat broths to produce nourishing and flavorful soups and sauces has almost completely disappeared from the American culinary tradition. Properly prepared, meat stocks are extremely nutritious, containing the minerals of bone, cartilage, marrow and vegetables as electrolytes, a form that is easy to assimilate. Adding wine or vinegar during cooking helps to draw minerals, particularly calcium, magnesium, and potassium, into the broth.

Dr. Francis Pottenger, author of the famous cat studies as well as articles on the benefits of gelatin in broth, taught that the stockpot was the most important piece of equipment to have in one's kitchen. It was Dr. Pottenger who pointed out that stock is also of great value because it supplies hydrophilic (water-loving) colloids to the diet. Raw food compounds are colloidal and tend to be hydrophilic, meaning that they attract liquids. Thus when we eat a salad or some other raw food, the hydrophilic colloids attract digestive juices for rapid and effective digestion. Colloids that have been heated are generally hydrophobic (they repel liquids), making cooked foods harder to digest. However, the proteinaceous gelatin in meat broths has the unusual property of attracting liquids; it is hydrophilic, even after it has been heated. The same property by which gelatin attracts water to form desserts, like Jell-O, allows it to attract digestive juices to the surface of cooked food particles.

The public is generally unaware of the large amount of research on the beneficial effects of gelatin taken with food. Gelatin acts first and foremost as an aid to digestion and has been used in the treatment of many intestinal disorders, including hyperacidity, colitis, and Crohn's disease. Although gelatin is by no means a complete protein, containing only the amino acids arginine and glycine in large amounts, it acts as a protein sparer, allowing the body to more fully utilize the complete proteins that are taken in. Thus, gelatin-rich broths are a must for those who cannot afford large amounts of meat in their diets. Gelatin also seems to be of use in the treatment of many chronic disorders, including; anemia and other diseases of the blood, diabetes, muscular dystrophy, and even cancer. Other important ingredients that go into broth are the components of cartilage, which recently have been used with remarkable results in the treatment of cancer and bone disorders, and of collagen, used to treat rheumatoid arthritis and other ailments. In folk wisdom, gelatin-rich chicken broth—the famous Jewish penicillin—is a valued remedy for the flu. Modern research has confirmed that broth helps prevent and mitigate infectious diseases. The wise food provider who uses gelatin-rich broth on a daily or frequent basis provides continuous protection from any health problems. It's easy to use broths and still thrive in our fast-paced world.

Oral Bio-Identical HA

One of the most important discoveries in the HA field is the discovery of HA specific receptors (CD44) in the oral cavity and throat that absorb bio-identical or HMW HA. Knowing how a substance gets into the body is key to getting its benefits. What benefit would you get as a diabetic if you drank your insulin each day instead of injecting it? You could know everything else about insulin, but it wouldn't do your blood sugar any good because it would be digested in your stomach, rendering it useless to control your blood sugar levels. Similarly, other substances that are traditionally injected, but thought to work orally must have studies to show oral equivalency. A case in point is chondroitin sulfate.

When designing medicines that will be absorbed via the oral cavity, scientists first look for high compatibility between the lining of the mouth and the active ingredient itself. Often a carrier molecule must be used to enhance compatibility.

In this case, HA has a great advantage. The tissues that comprise the mucous membrane of the oral cavity are rich in high molecular weight (HMW) hyaluronic acid. When liquid HMW HA is put into the mouth, the lining recognizes the added HA and readily accepts it into the membrane.

This "absorption advantage" helps explain why lower dosages of liquid HA outperformed higher doses of HA in capsules and tablets. When we consider how capsules and tablets work, releasing their contents in the stomach and intestines, we see the problem with taking HA this way and expecting superior results. With these solid forms, the HA is released too late, after the vast majority of CD44 receptors in the oral cavity and throat have already been passed. In addition, most of these formulas use a lower weight HA, much more like the "spent," broken-down HA that the body discards.

Advantage of a Lozenge

It is well-known that only hyaluronic acid of high molecular weight (HMW) is active as an anti-inflammatory. For that reason, it is important to preserve the molecular weight and the activity of the HA molecule. When HMW HA (2.4 million +) Daltons reaches the stomach, it is broken down into smaller, less effective fragments by the acids secreted there. Indeed acid hydrolysis (the breaking of the chemical bond) is often used to analyze biopolymers in analytical experiments.

Following these simple guidelines and remembering to include HA in oral and topical forms (including shampoos, conditioners, moisturizers, lotions, and other delivery vehicles) will do so much for your inner health and outer beauty. The HA miracle is upon us. This is your a-HA moment. What are you waiting for?

9

Shopping for a Great HA Supplement

There are many HA products available now on the market, making your shopping choice all the more important. Indeed, we expect to see more innovative HA formulas well in the near future.

The most absorbable and reliable choice would be a high molecular weight HA, around the 2.4-3 million Daltons range, according to experts writing in 2004 in the *Journal of Applied Nutrition* who examined the different kinds available. The researchers note, "dietary supplements containing HA are not equivalent due to the inherent properties of the three major types of HA commercially available as dietary supplement materials. Consumers and health care professionals need to be aware of the different types of HA and their very large differences in properties (even before ingestion). One source, hydrolyzed chicken sternal cartilage, is clearly unlike native HA, does not match the biological properties of native HA, and consequently should not be represented as HA to consumers on product labels..." Ultimately, the researchers recommend bio-identical high-molecular weight HA, purified non-animal HA because it most closely resembles the substance found in the body. It is this HA that has powerful anti-aging and lubricating qualities. Now, go out and get young again with HA!

Resources

Be sure to seek bio-identical high molecular weight HA of non-animal origin. Our recommended formulas are available at all fine health food stores, natural lifestyle and quality online retailers.

References

Andrews GP, Laverty TP, Jones DS "Mucoadhesive polymeric platforms for controlled drug delivery." *Eur. J. Pharmaceutics and Biopharmaceutics* 71(3):505-518 (2009).

Aruffo A, Stamenkovic I, Meinick M, Underhill CB, Seed B "CD44 is the Principal Cell Surface Receptor for Hyaluronate Cell." *Cell* (61): 1303-1313 (1990).

Bosworth TR, Scott JE "A specific fluorometric assay for hexosamines in glycosaminoglycans, based on deaminative cleavage with nitrous acid." *Anal Biochem* 223(2):266-73 (1994).

Bouhamidi R, Prévost V, Nouvelot A "High protection by grape seed proanthocyanidins (GSPC) of polyunsaturated fatty acids against UV-C induced peroxidation." *C R Acad Sci III*, 321(1):31-8, 1998.

Bravetti G "Preventive medical treatment of senile cataract with vitamin E and anthocyanosides: clinical evaluation." *Ann Ottalmol Clin Ocul* 115:109, 1989.

Burton G, Ingold K "Beta-carotene: an unusual type of lipid antioxidant." *Science* 224:569-73, 1984.

Jacques PF, Chylack LT Jr, McGandy RB, et al. "Antioxidant status in persons with and without senile cataract." *Arch Ophthalmol*, 106(3):337-40, 1988.

Kawcak CE, Frisbie DD, Trotter GW, McIlwraith CW, Gillette SM, Powers BE, Walton RM "Effects of intravenous administration of sodium hyaluronate on carpal joints in exercising horses after arthroscopic surgery and osteochondral fragmentation" *Am J Vet Res* 58(10) 1132-40 (1997).

Lalenti, A, Di Rosa M "Hyaluronic Acid Modulates Acute and Chronic Inflammation." *Agents Actions* 43, 44-47 (1994).

Sobocinski PZ, Canterbury WJ, Jurgens KH "Improved continuous-flow method for determination of total serum hexosamines." *Clin Chem* 22(8):1394-6 (1976).

Taylor A "Cataract: Relationships between nutrition and oxidation." *J Am Coll Nutr* 12:138-46, 1993.

Washington K, Gottfried MR, Telen MJ "Expression of the cell adhesion molecule CD44 in gastric adenocarcinomas." *Hum Pathol* 25(10):1043-9 (1994).

Wright KE, Maurer SG, DiCesare PE "Viscosupplementation for osteoarthritis." *Am J Orthop* 29(2)18-89 (2000).

Xiang Q, Lee YY, Petterson PO, Robert W "Torget Heterogeneous aspects of acid hydrolysis of a-cellulose." *Applied Biochemistry and Biotechnology* Humana Press, Inc. 107(1-3) pp 505-521 Spring, 2003.

Index